STRENGTH TRAINING FOR SENIORS

A Blueprint for Senior Strength and Vitality

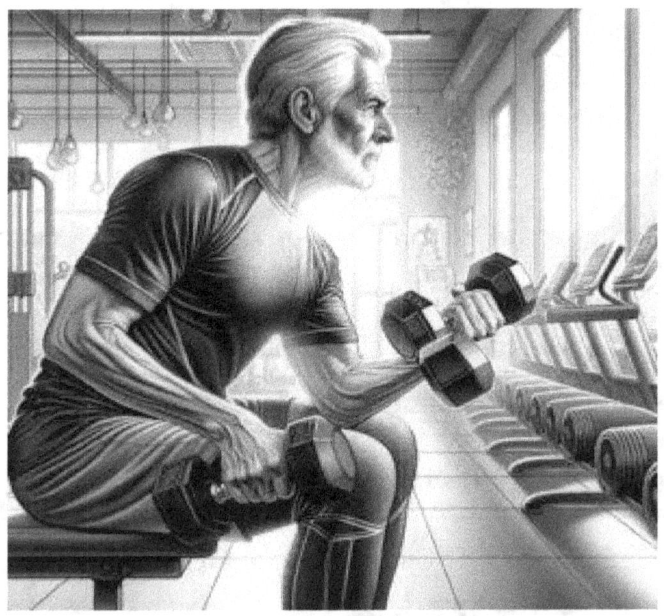

Desmond T. Hall

Copyright © 2024 by Desmond T. Hall

Declaimer

This book is a work of nonfiction. Names, characters, places, and incidents are either the product of the author's imagination or are used fictitiously. Any resemblance to actual persons, living or dead, business establishments, events, or locales is entirely coincidental.

OTHER FITNESS BOOKS BY THIS AUTHOR

Scan the QR Code Below to Get Access

TABLE OF CONTENTS

INTRODUCTIONS

Begin your path to recapture your energy and strength with "Strength Training for Seniors," a handbook designed to change the way you age. With each page, you'll be empowered to debunk age-related beliefs, paving the way to a stronger, more vibrant version of yourself. This is more than just a book; it is a revolution in senior fitness, designed to help you thrive in your golden years.

Why should you do strength training? Because the data is clear: regular strength training not only revitalizes your body, but it also sharpens your intellect, improves balance, and improves your entire quality of life. But where should you start? Right here. "Strength Training for Seniors" demystifies the method, making it understandable, reasonable, and, most importantly, possible for everyone.

This book will accompany you through each phase of your fitness journey. Every chapter is a step closer to a better, healthier you, from refuting myths, setting achievable objectives, and creating a tailored training plan that matches your lifestyle. You'll master the principles of strength training with workouts tailored to senior bodies, assuring safety and efficacy. Furthermore, we've added dietary and recuperation tips to supplement your physical efforts and maximize your outcomes.

However, "Strength Training for Seniors" is more than just a fitness guidebook; it's a source of incentive. It is about conquering the emotional and physical challenges that aging may provide, with the help of a community of like-minded people going on the same path. Whether you want to start a fitness adventure, improve your existing routine, or discover inspiration, this book is the first step toward becoming a stronger, more powerful person.

Let's defy age together, one rep at a time.

CHAPTER 1

The Importance of Strength Training in Aging

Our bodies naturally change as we age, which can have an impact on our physical ability and general quality of life. However, incorporating strength training into our fitness routine may considerably lessen these impacts, showing to be a foundation for aging with grace, strength, and vitality. The value of strength training in aging cannot be emphasized, as it provides several advantages that reach far beyond the walls of a gym.

First and foremost, strength training combats muscle loss (sarcopenia) and bone density decrease, two of the most significant aging-related alterations. After the age of 30, people can lose 3% to 5% of their muscle mass every decade, a pace that increases after the age of 60. This loss of muscle mass has an impact not only on physical strength and endurance, but also on metabolic health, raising the risk of chronic disorders including obesity, type 2 diabetes, and cardiovascular disease. Seniors who engage in regular physical workouts can keep and even develop muscle mass, which improves metabolism and insulin sensitivity.

Furthermore, strength training helps to preserve bone density. As we age, our bones gradually lose density, making them more weak and prone to fracture. Strength training promotes bone development and density, lowering the risk of osteoporosis and fractures, which are significant concerns among seniors. This bone and muscle fortification works together to enhance balance and coordination, considerably lowering the chance of falls, which are the primary cause of injury among the elderly.

Strength training also improves mental wellness and cognitive function. Exercise has been found to increase mood, alleviate symptoms of sadness and anxiety, and improve cognitive performance by stimulating neurogenesis—the formation of new brain cells. Regular strength exercise can assist elders retain mental clarity, increase memory, and promote general well-being.

Strength training can lead to better independence and quality of life in old age. Seniors who improve their strength, balance, and flexibility are better able to carry groceries, climb stairs, and play with grandkids. This autonomy is essential for retaining confidence and a positive self-image, resulting in a more active, engaged, and meaningful existence.

Strength training also promotes a sense of camaraderie and connection among seniors who attend group programs or gym sessions. This social engagement is essential for overcoming loneliness and isolation, fostering a sense of belonging, and improving overall happiness and lifespan.

Overcoming Common Myths and Fears

Beginning a strength training journey in your later years might be difficult, owing to numerous beliefs and worries about fitness for seniors. These myths might discourage older persons from engaging in strength exercise, despite its obvious advantages. Addressing and dispelling these stereotypes is critical for encouraging elders to begin the journey toward a healthier, more active lifestyle.

- **Myth 1: Strength training is not safe for older adults.**

One of the most common misconceptions is that strength training is inherently dangerous for seniors and poses a significant risk of injury. However, when done appropriately and under supervision, strength training is not only safe but also useful to older folks. It strengthens muscles and bones, lowers the chance of falls, and can help with symptoms of chronic illnesses including arthritis, diabetes, and heart disease. The idea is to begin with small weights and progressively raise the intensity under expert supervision.

- **Myth 2: It is too late to start.**

Many people assume that the advantages of exercise decline with age, however research regularly demonstrates that people of all ages can gain muscle and increase their fitness levels. Starting strength training later in age can still result in considerable health benefits, increased mobility, and improved quality of life. The body's ability for resilience and adaptation lasts throughout life, so any time is a good time to start.

- **Myth 3: Strength Training Makes Seniors Bulky.**

Another widespread worry is that strength training may result in excessive muscular mass. In actuality, growing a significant amount of muscle mass is difficult, especially for younger people, and necessitates precise, hard exercise regimens along with a focused diet. Strength exercise will help most seniors develop muscular tone and strength without adding mass, resulting in a leaner, healthier appearance.

- **Myth 4: Strength training isn't beneficial if you have chronic conditions.**

Many seniors with chronic diseases avoid strength training for fear of worsening their symptoms. On the contrary, strength training that is targeted to individual skills and requirements may be quite useful. It can aid with symptom management, improving insulin sensitivity in diabetes, improving cardiovascular health, and relieving arthritic pain and stiffness. Consulting with healthcare specialists can help guarantee a safe and successful strategy that is personalized to one's specific health state.

Fear of failure.

Fear of not being able to complete exercises correctly or not seeing results can be depressing. It is critical to set reasonable goals and recognize that development in strength training, like any other kind of exercise, is gradual. Celebrating little triumphs and constant work is more vital than quick outcomes.

Social Anxiety

Some seniors find the concept of exercising in a gym or group environment frightening. Beginning with home workouts or one-on-one sessions with a personal trainer might help you transition into the regimen more painlessly. Many people eventually discover that group lessons provide them with motivation and social support.

To overcome these beliefs and anxieties, education and support are essential. Learning about the benefits of strength exercise and distinguishing between facts and myths may help seniors take care of their own health. With adequate direction, a specific workout regimen, and a supportive atmosphere, strength training may be a safe, pleasurable, and fulfilling element of graceful aging.

Setting Realistic Fitness Goals

Setting realistic fitness objectives is essential for any effective strength training program, particularly for seniors commencing on their fitness journey. Goals not only give direction and purpose, but they may also be used to motivate people. However, the key to successful goal-setting is reality and flexibility to individual abilities, requirements, and lifestyles. For seniors, this entails accepting and appreciating the body's changes with age, focusing on functional fitness, and putting health and well-being ahead of aesthetic or competitive goals.

Understanding Your Starting Point.

Setting realistic fitness goals begins with an honest assessment of your present physical condition. This may entail speaking with a healthcare specialist or a fitness professional to assess your strength, flexibility, balance, and overall health. Recognizing pre-existing health concerns, such as arthritis, heart disease, or diabetes, is critical in developing a program that targets these illnesses without worsening them.

Define Success.

Success in a senior exercise program may differ from the goals set by younger folks. While muscular tone and strength gains are essential, for seniors, the emphasis frequently turns to improving quality of life. This might include creating objectives for improving balance to decrease fall risk, strengthening endurance for daily tasks, or managing chronic pain. Success can also be assessed in more subjective ways, such as feeling more energized, sleeping better, or experiencing a mood boost.

SMART Goals

The SMART framework is a useful tool for defining attainable objectives. It stands for specific, measurable, attainable, relevant, and time-bound. "I want to get stronger" is less effective than "I aim to increase my leg strength to complete five chair stands without assistance in eight weeks." The latter is explicit, quantifiable (number of chair stands), attainable (via progressive training), relevant (improves functional strength), and time-bound (eight weeks).

Incremental Progress

For seniors, particularly those who are new to exercising, setting modest, incremental objectives is critical. This method not only helps to avoid injury, but it also boosts confidence and enthusiasm. Incremental objectives make the process less intimidating and more achievable by establishing defined milestones and opportunities for celebration along the way.

Flexibility and Patience

The aging body reacts differently to exercise, so development may be slower or more variable than anticipated. It is critical to be flexible in your objectives, altering them as needed based on your body's responses and any external variables that may disrupt your routine, such as travel, sickness, or family obligations. Patience is essential; the advantages of strength training, while undeniable, might take time to materialize, particularly if you're starting from a low to no level of physical activity.

Holistic Goals

While strength training emphasizes physical health, setting objectives for mental and emotional well-being may be extremely useful. This might include goals like stress reduction, better sleep quality, or developing social ties through group fitness courses. A comprehensive approach guarantees that your fitness journey benefits every element of your life.

CHAPTER 2

Getting Started with Strength Training

Starting strength training may be a life-changing experience for elders, leading to better health, more mobility, and a greater sense of independence. This journey, while gratifying, sometimes starts with doubts and uncertainties. How does one begin? What safeguards are necessary? This section seeks to walk seniors through the first stages of starting a strength training program, stressing safety, pleasure, and the development of a routine that can be maintained over time.

Consulting with Healthcare Professionals.

The first, and possibly most important, step in establishing a strength training plan is to confer with healthcare experts. This is especially crucial for seniors who have pre-existing health concerns or have been physically inactive. A medical specialist may advise you on which workouts to prioritize or avoid, as well as suggestions for adaptations to meet any physical constraints. This guarantees that your strength training program not only helps you achieve your fitness objectives, but also improves your general health.

Understanding the fundamentals of strength training

At its heart, strength training consists of resistance-based workouts that increase muscular strength and endurance. This resistance can come from a variety of sources, including body weight, free weights such as dumbbells and barbells, resistance bands, and weight machines. For seniors just starting out, it's critical to become acquainted with these instruments and master the fundamentals of form and technique. Starting with body weight exercises or small weights is recommended to avoid the chance of injury and gradually increase strength.

Creating A Safe Exercise Environment

When first starting out with strength training, safety should be your main focus. This entails providing a safe workout environment, whether at home or at a gym. At home, make sure there's adequate space to move about without tripping risks. If you use a gym, make sure it has senior-friendly equipment and staff who can help and guide you. Regardless of the situation, having suitable footwear and comfortable clothing with a broad range of motion is vital.

Starting slowly and gradually

For seniors who are just starting out with strength training, the slogan "start slow and build gradually" cannot be emphasized enough. Initially, the emphasis should be on mastering the proper form for each exercise, even if it means using very little weights or none at all. Gradually increasing the weight or resistance over time helps the muscles to adapt, lowering the likelihood of strain or damage. It's also important to include a range of exercises that target different muscle groups to provide a well-rounded approach to strength training.

Incorporating Rest and Recovery

Rest and recuperation are equally crucial as the workouts themselves. Muscles require time to recover and strengthen, so getting enough rest in between workouts is essential. For seniors, this may mean beginning with strength training two to three times per week, with at least one day off in between. Listening to your body and avoiding pushing through pain is critical; discomfort is natural, but pain signals a need to pause and evaluate.

Seeking guidance and being motivated

For many seniors, advice from a fitness expert can be beneficial when starting a strength training program. A personal trainer with expertise dealing with older individuals can design exercises to your specific requirements and skills, ensuring that you complete them correctly and securely. Setting small, attainable objectives, as well as measuring progress over time, may also help keep motivation high. Remember that strength training is a journey with ups and downs, but the advantages to physical and mental health make the work worthwhile.

Beginning with strength training is a beneficial step toward a healthy and active aging process. Seniors may safely enjoy the numerous benefits of strength training by taking the necessary measures, mastering the basics, and progressively increasing the intensity of their exercises.

Preparing for Exercise: Safety First

Safety is the most important consideration for elders starting a strength training program. As we age, our bodies may become less robust, making it critical to take precautions to avoid injury and maintain a safe training environment. This section focuses on the critical steps elders should take before beginning an exercise regimen, incorporating the "safety first" idea to promote a healthy, long-term approach to fitness.

Consultation with healthcare professionals.

Before beginning any new fitness plan, talk with a healthcare expert. This phase is especially crucial for seniors who have pre-existing medical concerns including heart disease, arthritis, or diabetes. A healthcare provider may provide specific guidance on appropriate exercises and any precautions to ensure that your strength training program meets your health needs while remaining safe.

Self-awareness is important when preparing for exercise. Understand and heed your body's cues. If you feel pain or discomfort during a workout, it may be time to modify the activity or take a break. Understanding your present fitness level allows you to establish realistic objectives and choose routines that will not overstrain your ability.

Proper Warm-up and Cool-Down

A healthy warm-up prepares your body for increasing physical activity, which lowers the chance of injury. Warm-up exercises can comprise 5-10 minutes of light aerobic activity, such as walking or cycling, followed by dynamic stretches that resemble the motions used in strength training exercises. Cooling down is also vital, with mild stretching and relaxation activities to aid with muscle recovery and avoid stiffness.

Choosing the Right Equipment.

Choosing adequate workout equipment is critical for safety. Beginners should start with lesser weights and progressively increase resistance as their strength increases. Equipment should be comfortable to use and simple to hold, especially for people who have joint problems or arthritis. Resistance bands, lightweight dumbbells, and devices that allow for regulated motions are all terrific choices for seniors.

Safe environment and appropriate attire.

Make sure your training space is clear of risks that might cause trips and falls. Adequate room, proper lighting, and a non-slip floor are all crucial factors. Wearing adequate apparel is also important; comfortable, breathable clothes and supportive shoes improve safety and performance during exercise.

Learning proper form and techniques.

Strength training requires proper form and technique to be successful and avoid injuries. Incorrect form can cause strains, sprains, and more serious injuries. Beginners might consider working with a fitness expert or physical therapist to develop proper workout technique. Many community centers and gyms offer lessons for elders, offering a secure atmosphere for learning and practicing under expert supervision.

Listen to Your Body

One of the most essential safety precautions is to listen to your body. It is critical to distinguish between the natural discomfort of starting a new fitness plan and pain that indicates injury. Adjusting your training to fit how you feel on any given day is a practical way to stay healthy and active while avoiding injury.

Hydration and Nutrition

Staying hydrated and eating a healthy diet are essential for prepping for activity. Dehydration can cause dizziness and muscular cramps, limiting your ability to exercise safely. Similarly, good diet promotes muscle repair and energy levels, all of which are critical components of a successful strength training program for seniors.

Seniors who prioritize safety via these preparation procedures may comfortably engage in strength training, gaining its multiple advantages while reducing the danger of harm. This careful approach builds the groundwork for a fulfilling path to increased strength, mobility, and general well-being.

Understanding Your Body's Needs

Seniors who want to become healthier and stronger via strength training must first understand their body's specific demands. As we become older, our physical skills and health concerns alter, needing a personalized fitness regimen that takes these changes into account. Recognizing and adjusting to your body's signals is more than simply avoiding injury; it's about developing a long-term, efficient workout regimen that improves your quality of life.

Recognize physical limitations.

The first step in knowing your body's demands is to recognize any physical restrictions. These might be the result of chronic illnesses such as arthritis, osteoporosis, or heart disease, or just the natural decline in flexibility, balance, and muscle mass that occurs with age. Recognizing these constraints does not imply accepting them. Instead, it allows you to modify activities such that they improve your body without causing injury.

The significance of flexibility and balance

Flexibility and balance are important aspects of a senior's exercise regimen that are sometimes disregarded in favor of strength. However, these components are interrelated. Stretching exercises can help improve flexibility and range of motion, making strength training more effective and less likely to cause injury. Similarly, integrating balancing exercises helps reduce falls, which are a significant worry among older persons. Tai chi and easy balancing routines may be included into your regimen to improve general fitness and well-being.

Adapting To Energy Levels

Energy levels can vary greatly among seniors, depending on factors such as sleep quality, food, and mental health. Listen to your body and adjust your workout intensity accordingly. On days when you're feeling energized, you could try more difficult exercises or add an extra set to your workout. On low-energy days, concentrating on lighter activities or emphasizing rest may be more effective. This adaptable strategy guarantees that you satisfy your body's requirements without overexertion.

Hydration and Nutrition

Hydration and nutrition are critical in meeting your body's demands, particularly while strength training. Seniors may have a decreased feeling of thirst, increasing their risk of dehydration, which can impair muscular performance and recovery. Adequate hydration intake is critical before, during, and after exercise. A balanced diet high in proteins, healthy fats, and carbs promotes muscle regeneration and provides the energy required for exercise. A nutritionist can assist you in developing a diet plan that is appropriate for your fitness goals and nutritional requirements.

Rest and Recovery.

Understanding your body's demands also entails acknowledging the value of rest and rehabilitation. Strength training generates micro-tears in muscle fibers, which require time to mend and strengthen. Without appropriate rest, the risk of injury rises, and the efficacy of your exercises declines. Integrating rest days into your workout routine and getting enough sleep every night are critical for maximum recovery and performance.

Consultation and Continuous Learning

Finally, remaining knowledgeable about your health and fitness is critical for knowing your body's demands. Regular check-ups with healthcare specialists will help you monitor your condition and adapt your exercise routine as needed. Additionally, consulting with exercise specialists who specialize in senior fitness can give helpful insights into adapting your routine to your specific needs.

By using a holistic approach to understanding your body's demands, you can design a strength training program that not only tackles your physical limits and improves your overall health, but also brings pleasure and energy into your golden years. This individualized method guarantees that your path to strength and wellbeing is both safe and rewarding.

Essential Equipment for Home Workouts

Home exercises are quite convenient for seniors starting out on a strength training adventure. For people who are hesitant to navigate busy gyms, exercising at home provides flexibility, solitude, and a secure setting. However, constructing an efficient home gym does not need costly equipment or large rooms. This section discusses the needed equipment for senior-specific home workouts, with an emphasis on adaptability, safety, and efficiency.

Resistance Bands

Resistance bands are among of the most adaptable and senior-friendly pieces of equipment. They come in a variety of resistance levels, allowing for steady growth and adaptability according on your strength level. Bands may be used for a variety of workouts that target different muscular areas, including the arms, legs, and core. Their flexibility creates a unique resistance that mimics normal muscle activity, lowering the chance of damage. Furthermore, resistance bands are lightweight, inexpensive, and simple to store, making them excellent for home exercises.

Resistance training band

Dumbbells

Dumbbells are a classic in strength training, allowing you to execute a variety of exercises with just one set. Seniors should begin with lightweight dumbbells and progressively increase the weight as their strength develops. Choose dumbbells with ergonomic handles and non-slip surfaces to improve safety and comfort. Adjustable dumbbells, while somewhat more expensive, may be a space-saving and cost-effective alternative by allowing you to modify the weight based on your fitness level.

Dumbbells

Stability Ball

A stability ball may help you strengthen your core muscles *Stability ball* while also improving balance and posture. Exercises with a stability ball may be tailored to different fitness levels, making it a fantastic tool for both beginners and experienced users. It may also be used as a chair to improve core strength and balance while you're not exercising. To preserve perfect form throughout workouts, make sure you select the appropriate ball size for your height.

Yoga Mat

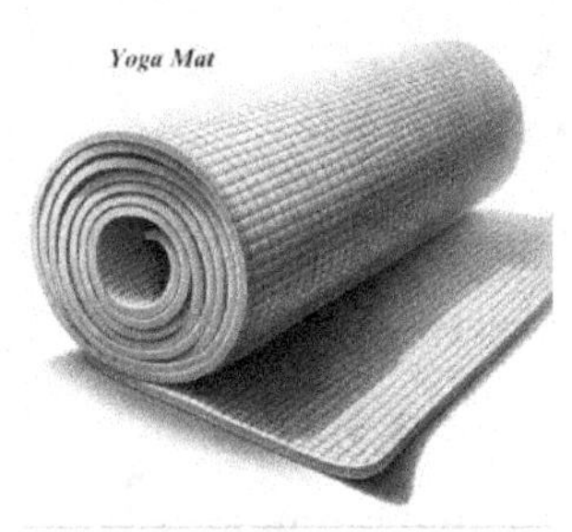

Yoga Mat

A yoga mat is vital for floor exercises that require cushioning and support, such as yoga, Pilates, stretching, and core workouts. The mat's nonslip surface helps to minimize slips and falls, making activities safer, particularly for people with balance issues. Furthermore, a high-quality yoga mat helps minimize joint strain during activities, increasing comfort and encouraging longer, more pleasurable workouts.

Chair

Flexibility exercise chair

A solid chair with no arms may be an essential piece of furniture for elders. It may be used for sitting workouts, which are ideal for beginners or those who have mobility limitations, as well as to assist balance and strength activities. Make sure the chair is firm and built of a robust material so it can securely support your weight during exercise.

Step Platform

A step platform is a simple method to include cardio into your weight training regimen, therefore boosting cardiovascular fitness and endurance. It is also suitable for strength workouts such as step-ups, which improve leg strength and balance. Choose a platform with a non-slip surface and adjustable height to vary the intensity of your workouts as your fitness increases.

Note Equipping your house for exercises does not necessitate a big investment of space or money. You can build a versatile and successful home gym with only a few important pieces of equipment, including resistance bands, dumbbells, a stability ball, a yoga mat, a solid chair, and a step platform. This system makes strength training accessible, pleasurable, and safe, allowing seniors to maintain and increase their fitness levels from the comfort of their own homes.

CHAPTER 3

Fundamental Strength Exercises for Seniors

For seniors starting out in strength training, learning foundational exercises is critical to laying a firm foundation for health. These exercises are intended to improve strength, balance, and flexibility, leading to a higher quality of life and greater independence. Here, we look at fundamental strength exercises designed specifically for seniors, stressing safety, efficacy, and the ability to execute them at home with minimum equipment.

1. Squats (Chair Squats)

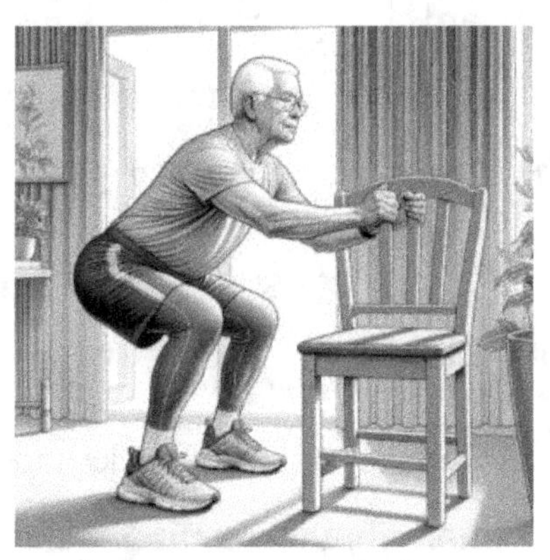

Squats are great for strengthening your legs, hips, and core, which is essential for everyday tasks like rising up from a chair or ascending stairs. Chair squats are a good place to start for novices or anyone who struggle with balance. Begin by standing in front of a chair, feet hip-width apart, then gently lowering yourself until seated, then standing back up. As your strength develops, attempt squats without sitting down, keeping a chair nearby for support if necessary.

2. Wall Push-ups

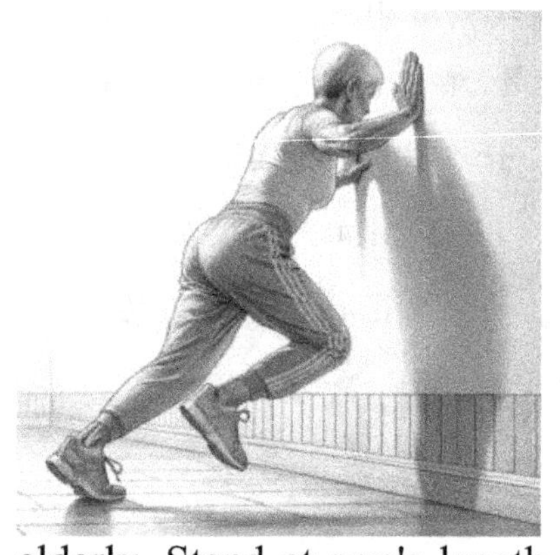

Push-ups work the upper body, particularly the chest, shoulders, and arms, which are essential for pushing doors and rising up from the floor. Wall push-ups are a milder variety suitable for elderly. Stand at arm's length from a wall, with your feet shoulder-width apart. Lean forward and place your palms against the wall, then push yourself back to the starting position. This exercise may be developed to counter push-ups and then standard push-ups on the floor.

3. Seated Row with Resistance Bands.

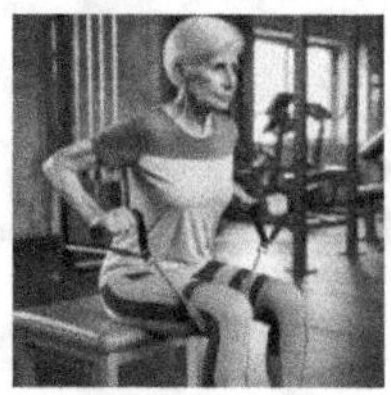

This workout focuses on the back and shoulders, improving posture and relieving back discomfort. Sit in a chair, feet flat on the ground, and grip a resistance band with both hands. Secure the band beneath your feet or around a solid item in front of you. Pull the band towards your waist, pressing your shoulder blades together, then gently let go. Control the movement by focusing on the muscles in your back and arms.

4. Leg Lifts.

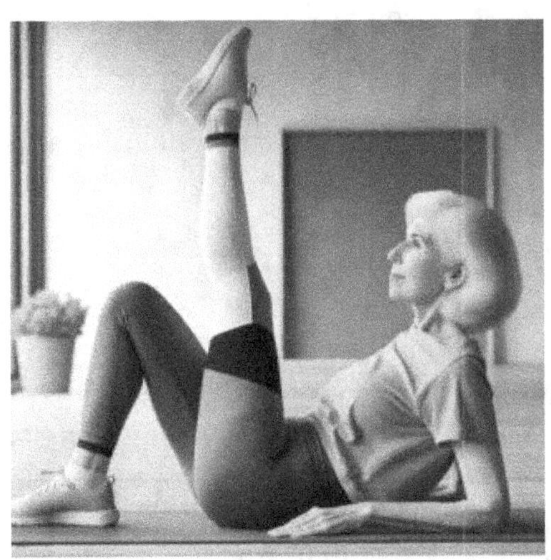

Leg lifts strengthen the thighs and increase hip flexibility, which is essential for mobility and balance. Lying on your side, elevate your upper leg to the ceiling while maintaining it straight, then drop it back down. This exercise may also be done while sitting by elevating one leg to the front or side without bending the knee. Ankle weights can provide additional resistance.

5. Toestands

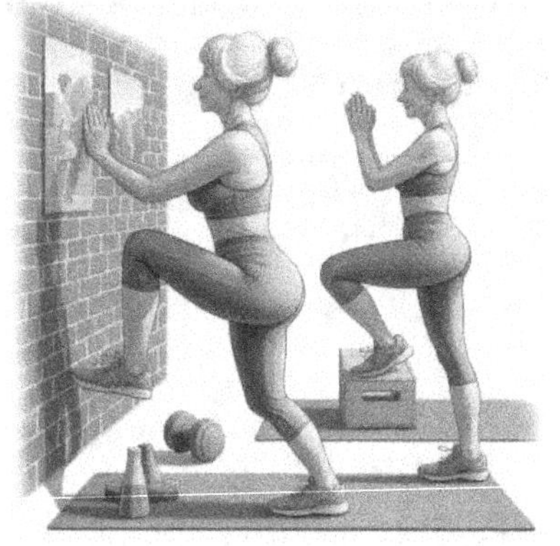

Toe stands or calf raises assist develop the lower leg muscles, which are necessary for walking and balancing. Holding onto a chair for support, carefully raise onto your toes and then descend back down. This exercise may be done standing or sitting, and it is very useful for strengthening ankle stability and lowering the chance of falling.

6. Bicep curls.

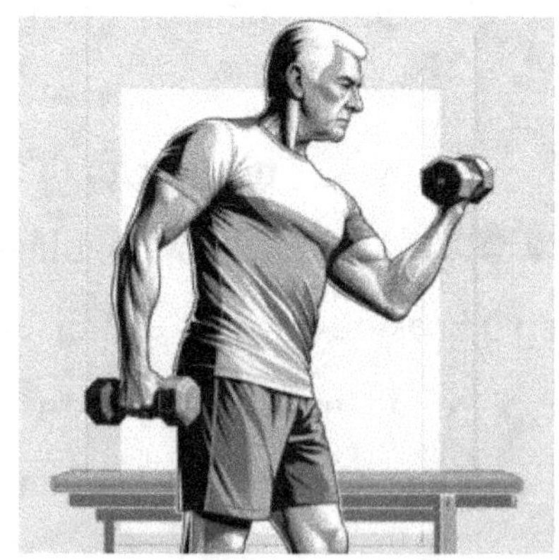

Strong arms are required for lifting and carrying goods, and bicep curls are an essential workout for doing this. Hold light dumbbells or a resistance band with palms facing up and elbows close to your body. Curl the weights towards your shoulders before slowly lowering them back down. Slow and controlled action, with a concentration on the biceps.

Including these essential exercises in a regular strength training regimen can have a major influence on seniors' physical health and general well-being. Each exercise focuses on important muscle areas needed for daily tasks, increasing independence and lowering the chance of falls and accidents. As always, listen to your body and speak with a healthcare expert before beginning any new fitness program to ensure that each activity is done safely and successfully. With regularity and perseverance, these essential activities can establish the framework for a healthier, more active senior life.

Upper Body Strength Essentials

Upper body strength is essential for preserving independence and doing everyday duties efficiently. Developing this area in seniors can dramatically improve their quality of life by enhancing functioning, balance, and general health. Here's a step-by-step guide to key upper body strength exercises for seniors, complete with safety and efficacy guidelines.

1. Wall Push-ups

Wall push-ups are a safer alternative to standard push-ups, putting less strain on the wrists and shoulders.

- Step 1: Stand facing a wall, about an arm's length away, with your feet shoulder-width apart.
- Step 2: Position your hands on the wall at shoulder height and breadth.
- Step 3: Keeping your torso straight, bend your elbows and drop your chest towards the wall.
- Step 4: Return to the beginning posture by extending your arms. Perform 10-15 reps.

2. Seated Overhead Press.

This workout focuses the shoulders and arms, which are essential for carrying items above.

- Step 1: Sit on a solid chair with no arms, holding a dumbbell in each hand at shoulder level, palms facing forward.
- Step 2: Raise the dumbbells until your arms are completely stretched without locking your elbows.

- Step 3: Lower the dumbbells to shoulder level. Aim for 8 to 12 repetitions.

3. Bicep curls.

Bicep curls strengthen the front region of the upper arms, which helps with lifting tasks.

- Step 1: Sit or stand with your back straight, gripping a dumbbell in each hand, arms outstretched, palms facing front.
- Step 2: With your elbows close to your torso, curl the weights towards your shoulders.
- Step 3: Slowly drop the dumbbells back to their starting position. Complete 10 to 15 repetitions.

4. Tricep Extension

Tricep extensions work the rear of the arms, which is essential for pushing actions.

- Step 1: Sit or stand with a dumbbell held above and arms straight.
- Step 2: Bend your elbows near to your head, then lower the dumbbell behind your head.

- Step 3: Extend your arms and hoist the weight back overhead. Perform 8 to 12 repetitions.

5. Seated rows using resistance bands.

Seated rows strengthen and enhance posture.

- Step 1: Sit on the floor, legs outstretched and back erect. Loop a resistance band around the soles of your feet, holding one end in each hand.
- Step 2: With your arms outstretched, pull the band toward your waist while bending your elbows and pushing your shoulder blades together.
- Step 3: Slowly return to your starting posture. Aim for 10 to 15 repetitions.

6. Chest press using resistance bands.

The chest press works the chest muscles and improves upper-body strength.

- Step 1: Place a resistance band at breast height behind you (for example, a closed door).
- Step 2: To produce tension, step forward while holding the ends of the band. Begin with arms bent at a 90-degree angle and elbows at chest level.

- Step 3: Push your arms forward until they are straight and at chest level.
- Step 4: Return to your starting position with control. Complete 8 to 12 repetitions.

Safety Tips:

Warm up your muscles before each workout with exercises like arm circles or shoulder shrugs.

Choose weights and resistance levels that allow you to complete each set with good technique while being demanding in the final few repetitions.

Breathe steadily throughout the exercises, exhaling on the exertion and inhaling on the return.

Incorporate rest days into your regimen to promote muscle repair and development.

Seniors who follow these carefully developed guidelines may safely increase their upper body strength, leading to a more active, independent, and rewarding existence.

Lower Body Strength Foundations

Lower body strength is essential for preserving balance, movement, and independence, particularly among seniors. Strengthening the muscles in the legs and hips aids with daily movements such as walking, climbing stairs, and getting up from a chair. This guide to core lower body workouts for seniors includes step-by-step directions to guarantee safety and efficacy.

1. Chair squats.

Chair squats strengthen the thighs and buttocks while improving balance.

- Step 1: Stand in front of a sturdy chair, feet hip-width apart and toes slightly pointing out.
- Step 2: Extend your arms in front of you to maintain balance.
- Step 3: Slowly bend your knees and lower yourself towards the chair, as if you are going to sit down.
- Step 4: Gently contact the chair with your buttocks before pushing through your heels to stand back up. Perform 10-15 reps.

2. Standing leg curls.

This workout focuses the hamstrings, which are essential for knee stability.

- Step 1: Stand behind a chair, holding onto its back for support.
- Step 2: Bend one knee slowly, lowering your heel as far towards your buttocks as is comfortable.
- Step 3: Hold the posture for a time before lowering your foot back to the floor. Perform 10-15 repetitions with each leg.

3. Side-Leg Raises

Side leg raises strengthen the hips and outer thighs, which are essential for side-to-side motions.

- Step 1: Stand behind a chair, holding onto its back for balance.
- Step 2: Keep your torso straight and elevate one leg to the side with your toe pointed front.
- Step 3: Lift the leg as high as is comfortable without tilting your torso, then drop it back down. Aim for 10-15 reps per side.

4. Toestands

Toe stands increase calf strength and ankle stability, which improves walking and balance.

- Step 1: Stand behind a chair, holding onto its back for support.

- Step 2: Gradually climb to your tiptoes, as high as possible.

- Step 3: Hold the position for a second before slowly lowering your heels back to the floor. Perform 10-15 reps.

5. Seated Knee Extensions.

Knee extensions aim to strengthen the quadriceps, which are essential for knee health and stability.

- Step 1: Sit in a chair, feet flat on the ground and back straight.

- Step 2: Extend one leg at a time and straighten it in front of you.

- Step 3: Hold the stretched position for a few seconds before slowly lowering your foot back to the floor. Complete 10-15 repetitions for each leg.

6. Seated Hip Marching

This exercise works the hip flexors and thighs, increasing mobility.

- Step 1: Settle into a chair with your feet flat on the floor and your back straight.
- Step 2: Lift one knee as high as you can while keeping the other foot on the ground.
- Step 3: Maintain the position for a second before lowering your leg back down. Alternate legs, repeating 10-15 times on each side.

Safety Tips:

1. Start each exercise session with a warm-up, such as easy marching in place, to prepare your muscles and joints.
2. Choose a chair that is solid and does not slip or tip over easily.
3. Wear supportive shoes to offer a solid foundation and avoid slipping.
4. Listen to your body and adjust routines to meet any discomfort or limits.

Incorporating these basic lower-body exercises into a daily workout program will help seniors improve their strength, balance, and general mobility. Always prioritize form and safety, and get advice from a healthcare expert before beginning a new workout program.

Core Stability and Flexibility

Core stability and flexibility are critical components of any well-rounded exercise regimen, particularly for seniors. A strong, stable core improves balance and posture, lowering the danger of falling, whereas flexibility helps preserve joint range of motion, making everyday tasks easier and minimizing the probability of injury. Here's a guide to exercises that enhance core stability and flexibility, specifically intended for seniors.

Core Stability Exercises

1. Sitting Belly Breathing

This workout uses regulated breathing to develop the deep core muscles.

- Step 1: Sit comfortably in a chair, feet flat on the floor, hands on your abdomen.

- Step 2: Inhale deeply through your nose, feeling your belly expand beneath your hands.

- Step 3: Exhale gently through your lips, squeezing your abdominal muscles and bringing your belly button towards your spine.

- Step 4: Take 10-15 breaths, focusing on deep, controlled movements.

2. Seated leg lifts.

Leg lifts work the lower abdominal muscles and enhance core stability.

- Step 1: Sit on the edge of a chair, back straight and hands resting on it for support.

- Step 2: Keeping one leg straight, carefully elevate it off the ground as high as is comfortable.

- Step 3: Maintain the posture for a few seconds before lowering the leg back down.

- Step 4: Repeat for the opposite leg. Perform 10-15 reps per leg.

3. Chair Plank.

This modified plank exercise targets the whole core without requiring you to go down on the floor.

- Step 1: Stand facing the back of a solid chair and place your hands on its back.
- Step 2: Move back until your body creates a straight line from your head to your heels, similar to the plank posture.
- Step 3: For 20-30 seconds, hold this position with your core engaged.
- Step 4: Take a rest and repeat 2-3 times.

Flexibility Exercises: 1. Seated Toe Touch.

This exercise stretches the hamstrings and lower back, which increases flexibility.

- Step 1: Sit on the edge of a chair, legs outstretched and heels on the floor.
- Step 2: Extend your arms towards your toes, then bend forward by hinging at the hip.
- Step 3: Reach as far as you feel comfortable, attempting to touch your toes, and hold for 15-30 seconds.
- Step 4: Gradually sit back up. Repeat 2–3 times.

2. Chest Opener.

This stretch increases flexibility in the chest and shoulders, resulting in better posture.

- Step 1: Stand or sit with your back straight.
- Step 2: Clasp your hands behind your back and straighten your arms.
- Step 3: Gently raise your hands and press your chest forward, experiencing a stretch in your shoulders and chest.
- Step 4: Hold for 15-30 seconds and then release. Repeat 2–3 times.

3. Upper Back Stretch

This exercise extends the upper back and shoulders, which relieves stress.

- Step one: Sit or stand with your back straight.
- Step 2: Reach out your arms in front of you and clasp your hands together.
- Step 3: Push your hands forward, rounding your upper back and tucking your chin slightly.

- Step 4: Hold the stretch for 15-30 seconds while feeling the stretch between your shoulder blades.
- Step 5: Release and repeat 2-3 times.

Including these core stability and flexibility exercises in your training program will improve your overall health and mobility. Always move slowly and deliberately, inhaling deeply and focusing on form. If any workout causes pain or discomfort, discontinue immediately and check with a doctor. With consistent practice, these exercises can help maintain and even enhance core strength and flexibility, resulting in a more active and independent lifestyle.

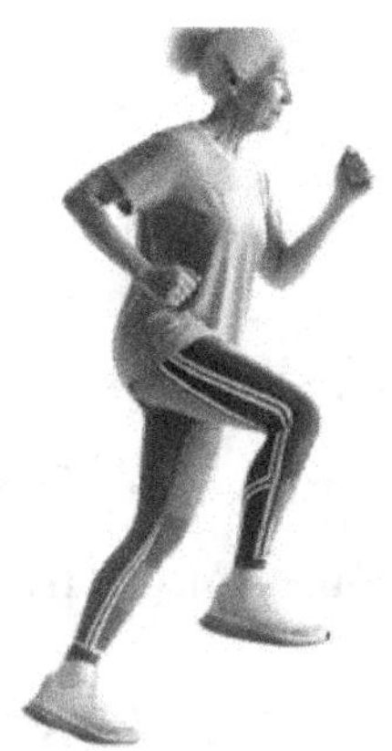

CHAPTER 4

Designing Your Strength Training Routine

Designing a strength training plan for seniors necessitates careful consideration of a number of important elements, including personal health state, fitness objectives, and exercise science concepts. A well-structured program not only increases the advantages of strength training, but it also reduces the chance of injury, resulting in a safe and effective method to enhancing physical health and overall wellness. This is a complete guide on creating a specific strength training plan for seniors.

Understanding Your Starting Point.

Begin by examining your existing fitness level, health status, and physical limits. Consult a healthcare expert to acquire clearance for exercise and to address any specific concerns. This first examination will assist in tailoring your routine to your talents and goals, guaranteeing safety and efficacy.

Setting Realistic Goals.

Determine clear, attainable goals based on your assessment. Your goals, whether they be to improve balance, muscle strength, flexibility, or all of the above, should be precise, measurable, achievable, relevant, and time-bound (SMART). This clarity will help you arrange your routine and stay motivated.

Balancing the components.

A thorough strength training regimen for seniors should include exercises that target all main muscle groups, including upper and lower body, core, and flexibility work. Incorporating a variety of these components enables a comprehensive strategy that improves overall fitness without stressing any specific area.

1. Upper-Body Strength

Include workouts for the arms, shoulders, chest, and back. Examples include wall push-ups, seated overhead presses, and bicep curls. These workouts help you do daily chores like carrying groceries and reaching above.

2. Lower-Body Strength

Chair squats, leg lifts, and toe stands are all workouts that will help to strengthen your legs and hips. Strong legs and hips are essential for maintaining balance while walking and climbing stairs.

3. Core Stability.

Incorporate exercises that improve core strength and stability, such as sitting belly breathing or chair planks. A strong core promotes proper posture and lowers the chance of falling.

4. Flexibility

Stretching activities can help increase flexibility and range of motion. Flexibility exercises can be included in the warm-up or cool-down phases, with a focus on main muscle groups and joints.

Frequency and Volume

For seniors, starting with two to three strength training sessions per week on non-consecutive days is advised. This frequency ensures proper recuperation while also boosting strength increases. Each session should have 8-10 exercises that target the major muscular groups, with 1-3 sets of 10-15 repetitions each. The volume may be modified to suit individual endurance and strength levels.

Progress and Adaptation

Gradually raise the intensity of your workouts as you gain strength. This can be accomplished by raising the weight, repetitions or sets, or integrating more difficult exercises. To minimize overexertion, advancement should be steady and controlled, with an emphasis on listening to your body's cues.

Monitoring and Adjusting

Regularly evaluate your progress toward your goals and change your regimen as appropriate. This might include changing workouts, adjusting the intensity, or addressing any new health issues that occur. Flexibility in your approach enables for long-term improvement while also keeping your strength training regimen interesting and engaging.

Safety and enjoyment

Safety should always be a concern. Use appropriate form, begin with modest weights, and focus on activities that do not cause discomfort or agony. Choose activities that you love in order to make your strength training regimen not only healthy but also enjoyable and satisfying.

By adhering to these rules, seniors may create a strength training plan that is safe, pleasant, and suited to their own fitness demands and goals. This tailored approach promotes physical health, improves quality of life, and fosters independence in the senior years.

Creating a Balanced Workout Plan

A balanced training routine is vital for seniors who want to improve their strength, flexibility, and general health. A well-rounded regimen integrates a variety of exercise disciplines to provide holistic advantages such as greater muscle strength, balance, flexibility, and cardiovascular health. Here's how seniors may create a balanced training regimen that is tailored to their specific requirements and goals.

1. Evaluate fitness levels and goals.

Begin by assessing your current fitness and health state. Consider any current health issues or physical restrictions. Setting specific, attainable objectives is critical, whether it's to gain muscle strength, balance, flexibility, or stamina. Understanding where you are and where you want to go will help shape the structure of your training plan.

2. Implement strength training.

Strength training should be a key component of your workout routine, with emphasis on major muscular groups such the legs, hips, back, abdomen, chest, shoulders, and arms. Use safe and effective workouts for seniors, such as chair squats, wall push-ups, and seated leg lifts. Aim for 2-3 days a week, with rest days in between to allow muscle recovery.

3. Add Balance Exercises.

Balance exercises are essential for preventing falls, a significant worry among seniors. Include balance-building activities such as standing on one foot, walking heel to toe, and tai chi. These exercises may be incorporated into your everyday practice to improve stability and coordination without requiring additional equipment.

4. Include flexibility in work.

Flexibility exercises assist to maintain the range of motion in your joints, making daily tasks simpler and lowering the chance of injury. Stretch main muscle groups on a regular basis, with an emphasis on mild stretching exercises that may be done every day. Yoga and Pilates are great for increasing flexibility and may be tailored to a variety of fitness levels.

5. Prioritize cardiovascular activities.

Cardiovascular exercise promotes heart health and stamina. Walking, swimming, and cycling are low-impact sports that seniors may do almost every day of the week. Begin with shorter periods, aiming for at least 150 minutes of moderate-intensity aerobic activity spaced out across the week, as advised by health standards.

6. Prepare for recovery.

Recovery is a crucial component of any training program, particularly for seniors. Incorporate rest days into your schedule to help your body recuperate and avoid overtraining. Listen to your body—if you're tired or sore, take extra rest or engage in milder exercises such as walking or moderate stretching.

7. Maintain flexibility and adjust as needed.

Your fitness levels and goals may vary over time, so you should evaluate and alter your training routine on a regular basis. Be willing to attempt new activities or change the intensity and frequency of your workouts in order to keep pushing your body and working toward your objectives.

8. Consult professionals.

Seek assistance from fitness professionals or healthcare specialists, particularly if you are starting a new exercise regimen or have pre-existing health issues. They may make tailored recommendations and guarantee that your training routine is safe and successful.

9. Enjoy the process.

Choose activities that you like to ensure that your training routine is both healthy and fun. Including a variety of activities in your program will keep things interesting and help you stay motivated over time.

A varied training regimen for seniors should include strength, balance, flexibility, and cardiovascular activities. Tailoring the plan to each individual's goals, preferences, and health state guarantees that seniors may improve their physical health and quality of life while reducing their risk of injury. Regular plan review and adaption will aid in the maintenance of progress and the engagement and effectiveness of workout routines.

Scheduling Your Workouts for Success

Workout scheduling is an important part of any effective fitness regimen, particularly for seniors. A well-planned timetable not only assures a balanced approach to training, but it also aids in consistency, energy management, and meeting long-term fitness objectives. Here's how seniors may successfully organize their workouts while taking into account the particular requirements and obstacles that come with age.

Understanding your body's rhythms

First, you need to understand your body's natural cycles. Seniors can notice that their energy levels fluctuate throughout the day. Some people feel more enthusiastic in the morning, while others find their groove later in the day. Listen to your body and plan your exercises when you're at your peak alertness and energy. This will allow you to perform better and enjoy your workouts more.

Balancing several types of exercises.

A well-balanced fitness routine for seniors should incorporate strength training, balancing exercises, flexibility routines, and cardiovascular activities. To minimize overexertion and allow for proper recuperation time, it is best to rotate between these sorts of workouts throughout the week. For example, you may arrange strength training on Mondays and Thursdays, balance and flexibility on Tuesdays and Fridays, and mild cardiovascular activities like walking or swimming on Wednesdays and weekends.

Incorporating Rest and Recovery

Rest and recuperation are equally crucial as the workouts themselves. Seniors should schedule one to two complete rest days every week to allow their bodies to heal. Consider scheduling milder activity days following more intensive workouts. This technique helps to minimize injury and tiredness, allowing you to stay on track with your fitness objectives over time.

Plan for Consistency.

Consistency is essential for reaching and sustaining fitness results. To build a habit, plan your workouts for the same time every day. This consistency helps to establish exercise as a habit, making it a natural part of your daily routine. If you like group courses or working out with a friend, scheduling them ahead of time might help you stay motivated and accountable.

Adjusting for energy and engagement.

Be prepared to change your schedule depending on how you feel. If you're having a day with little energy or motivation, it may be more useful to replace a scheduled high-intensity workout with something less taxing, such as a moderate yoga session or a walk. Listening to your body and being flexible with your schedule will help you keep a positive attitude toward exercise and prevent burnout.

Setting realistic timeframes

When organizing your workouts, be realistic about the amount of time you can devote to exercise. According to health standards, seniors should engage in at least 150 minutes of moderate aerobic exercise each week, as well as muscle-strengthening activities on two or more days of the week. Break this down into smaller chunks, remembering that even brief 10-15 minute workouts may be effective.

Including warm-up and cool-down.

Make sure your workout routine includes time for warm-up and cool-down. A decent warm-up prepares your body for activity and can help prevent injuries, whereas cooling down allows your body to return to a resting state, which reduces the chance of muscular discomfort.

Monitoring progress and making adjustments as needed.

Regularly assess and change your training program based on your success and how your body reacts to the workouts. This might include raising the intensity of your workouts, introducing new exercises, or slowing back if you're feeling fatigued or uncomfortable.

Seniors may achieve a balanced approach to fitness by carefully arranging workouts that fit into their lifestyle, optimize their health advantages, and provide the groundwork for long-term success in their fitness quest.

Progression and Adjusting Your Routine

For seniors starting out on a strength training adventure, scheduling sessions is a critical step in achieving fitness objectives. A well-planned timetable not only assures a balanced approach to exercise, but it also encourages consistency, safety, and enjoyment. Here's how seniors should carefully organize their training regimens for success, taking into account the special needs that come with age.

Start with realistic planning.

Begin by evaluating your present lifestyle, obligations, and energy levels during the day. Realistic planning is selecting training times when you feel the most energized and can regularly devote time to exercise. Many seniors like to do this in the morning when they have more energy, but others prefer the afternoon or early evening. The key is consistency; scheduling workouts at the same times each week might help build a pattern.

Balance your workout types.

Seniors should have a balanced fitness plan that includes strength training, aerobic activity, balancing activities, and flexibility exercises. Spread out these workouts throughout the week to minimize overexertion on any given day and to allow for muscle recovery, particularly following strength training sessions. For example, you may plan strength training on Mondays and Thursdays, cardiovascular activities on Tuesdays and Fridays, and balance and flexibility exercises on Wednesdays and Saturdays.

Incorporate Rest and Recovery.

Recovery is just as important as the activity itself, especially for seniors. Make sure your program includes rest days so your body can recuperate and adjust to the activities. Recovery might also include gentler exercise days, such as easy walking or yoga, which assist to sustain mobility without hurting the body.

Adjust for intensity and duration.

Workout intensity and length should be appropriate for your fitness level and goals. Begin with shorter, less intensive workouts, gradually increasing as your strength and endurance increase. A 30-minute strength training session may be a good beginning point, with incremental increases to 45-60 minutes as you gain confidence. Similarly, vary the intensity of cardiovascular activities according to your heart health and capabilities.

Plan for flexibility.

Life may be unpredictable, so a flexible workout program is necessary. Prepare a backup plan for days when your normal routine is not practical, such as shorter workouts at home or basic exercises that may be incorporated into everyday activities. This keeps you moving even when you can't stick to your set timetable.

Listen to your body.

Pay attention to how your body reacts to workouts. If you encounter unexpected discomfort or weariness, give yourself extra rest or consider reducing the intensity of your workouts. Listening to your body helps you avoid injuries and ensures that your training routine promotes your health and well-being.

Use tools and resources.

Consider using tools and services to help you plan and track your exercises. Calendars, apps, and even a basic notepad may all be useful for planning and tracking your progress. Some tools include reminders and motivating messages to help you stay on track.

Seek support.

Sharing your training routine with friends, family, or a fitness club may help you stay accountable and motivated. Others' encouragement and support might help you stick to your schedule and overcome obstacles.

Regularly review and adjust your schedule.

As you move through your fitness journey, your requirements and capacities may shift. Review your training routine on a regular basis and make any necessary adjustments to match your current fitness level, goals, and interests. This versatility guarantees that your exercises remain successful, pleasant, and consistent with your health and wellbeing goals.

Creating a workout routine that takes into account your particular preferences, fitness objectives, and physical limitations is critical for seniors' success in strength training and general health. By planning realistically, balancing workout styles, and listening to your body, you may create a long-term and pleasurable fitness regimen that supports your road to a healthier, more active lifestyle.

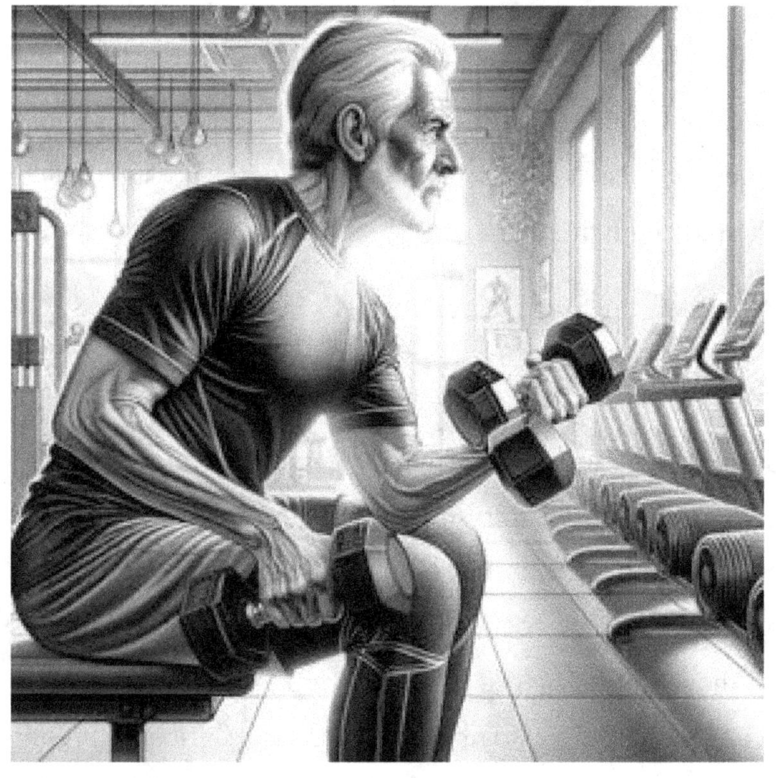

CHAPTER 5

Nutrition and Recovery for Senior Strength Training

Nutrition and recuperation are essential components of a thorough strength training program for seniors. As the body ages, it becomes increasingly important to eat appropriately and give enough recovery time in order to optimize the benefits of exercise, reduce injury risks, and promote general well-being. Here's a detailed look at how seniors may improve their diet and recovery techniques to supplement their strength training.

Nutrition for Strength Training.

1. Protein Intake.

Protein is essential for muscle repair and development, particularly following strength training sessions. Seniors require more protein than younger folks to maintain muscle growth, aid in recuperation, and maximize the effectiveness of their activities. Aim for a high-protein diet that includes lean meats, seafood, dairy, legumes, and plant-based protein sources. Incorporating protein into every meal and snack can assist satisfy these requirements, with a focus on ingesting protein after an exercise to aid with muscle repair.

2. A Balanced Diet

A well-balanced diet with a range of nutrients is vital for general health and strength training. Focus on consumption:

Carbohydrates offer energy during exercises. Whole grains, fruits, and vegetables are great sources.

Avocados, almonds, seeds, and olive oil include healthy fats, which are essential for joint health and vitality.

Vitamins and Minerals: A diet high in fruits, vegetables, lean meats, and whole grains provides a variety of vitamins and minerals essential for muscular function and recovery, such as calcium, vitamin D, magnesium, and potassium.

3. Hydration.

Staying hydrated is critical for older athletes because dehydration can impair muscular function and recovery. Water is the greatest option for staying hydrated. The amount required varies according to activity level, but aiming for at least 8 glasses of water each day is a good start.

Monitor your hydration levels by paying attention to thirst signals and urine color, aiming for light yellow.

Recovery Strategies:

- Ensure adequate rest: Rest days are essential in any strength training program, enabling muscles to recover and get stronger. Seniors, in particular, may require more recuperation time between sessions. Including rest days or light exercise days in your regimen might help your body recover and avoid overtraining.

- Quality sleep is essential for recuperation. During sleep, the body repairs muscle tissue and replenishes energy reserves. Aim for 7-9 hours of sleep every night, with a consistent sleep pattern to improve sleep quality and recovery.

3. Active Recovery.

Active rehabilitation is doing light, non-strenuous activities on rest days, such as walking, easy stretching, or yoga. These activities increase blood flow to muscles, which helps to relieve stiffness and speed up the healing process without overworking the body.

4. Stress Management.

Stress might impair the body's capacity to recuperate after exercise. Stress-reduction practices such as meditation, deep breathing exercises, and hobbies can all help with healing and well-being.

5. Listen to Your Body

Pay heed to the signs your body sends. If you feel extended pain, exhaustion, or other indicators of overexertion, take extra rest and check with a healthcare practitioner to verify your training and recovery procedures are suitable for your requirements.

For seniors who engage in strength training, balancing diet and recuperation is critical for optimizing exercise effects, stimulating muscle development and repair, and guaranteeing fitness longevity. Seniors may improve their strength, health, and lifestyle by focusing protein consumption, eating a balanced diet, staying hydrated, getting enough rest and sleep, and adopting active recovery and stress management.

Eating for Muscle Health and Energy

Eating for muscular health and vitality is critical, especially for seniors who participate in strength training. As we age, our systems become less effective at digesting nutrients and preserving muscle mass, so it's critical to eat a diet that promotes muscle repair, development, and overall energy levels. Here's a thorough guide to optimizing your nutrition for muscular health and long-term energy, specifically for seniors who participate in strength training programs.

Prioritize Protein

Muscles are made up of proteins. It is necessary for the healing of muscle tissues injured during strength training as well as the development of new muscle fibers. Seniors, in particular, require a greater protein intake to prevent age-related muscle loss (sarcopenia). Include a wide range of protein sources in your diet, including:

- Lean meats (chicken, turkey, and lean beef).
- Fish (particularly fatty fish such as salmon, which is also high in omega-3 fatty acids)
- Dairy items include milk, cheese, and yogurt.

- Plant-based proteins include beans, lentils, tofu, and quinoa.

Aiming for protein-rich snacks and meals throughout the day will help guarantee optimal intake, with an emphasis on ingesting protein within a 30-minute to 2-hour window after your strength training exercise to maximize muscle repair.

Embrace Healthy Carbohydrates

Your body and brain rely on carbohydrates as their major fuel source. Choosing the proper carbs is essential for staying energized throughout the day and throughout exercise. Choose complex carbs that offer a consistent flow of energy, such as:

- Whole grains (brown rice, oatmeal, and quinoa)
- Fruits and vegetables (particularly those rich in fiber)
- Legumes (beans, lentils)

These meals not only provide energy for everyday activity and exercise, but they also provide essential minerals and fiber that promote general health.

Include healthy fats.

Fats serve an important role in hormone manufacturing, particularly those required for muscle development and repair. To promote muscular health, include healthy fat sources in your diet, such as:

- Avocados Nuts and seeds.
- Olive oil, fatty seafood.

These fats also provide a concentrated supply of energy, allowing for sustained activity throughout the day.

Stay hydrated.

Hydration is needed for proper muscle function and energy. Water helps carry nutrients to your muscles and eliminate waste from your body. Dehydration can cause muscular cramps, weariness, and decreased performance. Aim for at least 8 glasses of water each day, or more if you're active or live in a hot environment. Monitoring the color of your urine is a useful sign of hydration; aim for pale yellow.

Vitamins and Minerals

Certain vitamins and minerals have specialized functions in muscle health and energy metabolism.

Ensure that your diet includes:

- Vitamin D and calcium promote bone health and muscular function.
- Magnesium helps muscles contract and relax.
- Iron for transporting oxygen to muscles.
- B vitamins promote energy generation.

These elements are normally obtained from a well-balanced diet rich in fruits and vegetables, whole grains, and lean meats. Seniors, on the other hand, may require additional vitamin D and calcium supplements if their food consumption is insufficient.

Timing is important.

The time of your meals might have an influence on your energy levels and muscular function. Eating modest, regular meals throughout the day will help you maintain a consistent energy level and a stable supply of nutrients to your muscles. Including protein and carbohydrate sources in your post-workout meal or snack can help with muscle healing and replenishing energy levels.

For seniors who focus on strength training, a diet that promotes muscular health and energy include prioritizing protein, selecting appropriate carbs and fats, staying hydrated, ensuring enough intake of critical vitamins and minerals, and considering meal time. Seniors who follow these nutritional rules can improve their muscular health, speed up recovery, and maintain high energy levels, all of which contribute to an active and healthy lifestyle.

The Role of Hydration in Fitness

Hydration is critical to seniors' general fitness and health, particularly for those who exercise often. Water is required for nearly every function in the body, including nutrition delivery, temperature control, and joint lubrication. Staying hydrated is critical for seniors who want to improve their workout performance, recover quickly, and maintain good health. Here's a closer look at the importance of water in exercise, especially for seniors.

Essential for Muscle Function

Muscles are made up of around 75% water, emphasizing the need of hydration for muscular function. Proper hydration contributes to the equilibrium of electrolytes, such as sodium and potassium, which are required for muscular contractions. Dehydration can cause muscular cramps, diminished strength, and endurance, reducing the efficiency of strength training exercises.

Improves joint lubrication.

Hydration is essential for keeping the joints adequately lubricated and flexible. Water helps to keep the synovial fluid flowing, which lowers friction and wear on joints during movement. Staying hydrated can assist seniors who are more prone to joint disorders avoid discomfort during exercise and daily activities, supporting a more active and pain-free existence.

Regulates body temperature.

During activity, the body's temperature rises, and water is necessary for thermoregulation. Sweating is the body's natural cooling mechanism, and appropriate fluid intake ensures that this process occurs efficiently, minimizing overheating. Seniors, in particular, may have a diminished capacity to control body temperature, making hydration more important during physical exertion.

Enhances Recovery

Hydration is essential for recovery following strength exercise. Water helps to carry nutrients to the muscles, which aids in healing and development. Furthermore, hydration helps to remove metabolic waste products produced during exercise, such as lactic acid, which can lead to muscular discomfort. Proper hydration can help lower the risk of delayed onset muscle soreness (DOMS) and speed up the healing process.

Supports cardiovascular health.

Hydration has a substantial impact on cardiovascular health, which influences exercise performance. Adequate fluid consumption helps to maintain blood volume, allowing the heart to pump blood more effectively and supply oxygen and nutrients to the muscles when exercising. For seniors, preserving cardiovascular health is critical for endurance and the capacity to engage in strenuous physical activity.

Cognitive Function and Energy Levels

Hydration affects cognitive function and energy levels. Even slight dehydration can impair concentration, memory, and mood, influencing motivation and focus during exercises.

Staying hydrated is critical for seniors to maintain mental clarity and maximize the cognitive health advantages of exercise.

Hydration Strategies for Seniors

Monitor fluid intake: Aim for at least 8 glasses of water every day, with adjustments based on activity level, environment, and personal needs.

- Include hydrating foods. Water-rich fruits and vegetables can help you stay hydrated.
- Monitor Hydration Status: Pay attention to thirst cues and the color of your urine, which should be light yellow.
- Balance Electrolytes: After a lengthy period of exertion, try drinking electrolyte-containing drinks to restore any losses caused by sweating.

Understanding the importance of water in fitness is critical for seniors who exercise for strength. Adequate hydration promotes muscular function, joint health, body temperature control, recuperation, cardiovascular health, and cognitive performance. Seniors can increase their physical performance, recuperation, and quality of life by using efficient hydration practices during ongoing exercise activities.

Rest and Recovery Strategies

Rest and recuperation are essential parts of any strength training program, particularly for seniors. These aspects are critical for allowing the body to repair and strengthen after exercise, lowering the chance of injury, and maintaining continuous fitness improvement. As seniors begin strength training, the necessity for good rest and recovery measures becomes even more apparent owing to the natural aging process, which can prolong recovery periods and increase susceptibility to injury. Here's a thorough guide on senior-specific rest and recovery practices.

Understanding the Importance of Rest

Rest days are essential in any strength training routine because they allow muscles to heal and develop stronger. Adequate rest days are necessary for seniors to avoid overuse injuries and allow for physiological adjustments. Seniors should allow at least one to two days of rest between sessions that target the same muscle areas to achieve full recovery.

Active Recovery

Active recuperation entails performing low-intensity activity on rest days. Walking, easy stretching, tai chi, and yoga can all aid to preserve mobility and blood circulation, making it easier to remove waste products produced in muscles during strength training. Active rehabilitation can help seniors not only heal physically, but also improve flexibility and balance, adding to overall well-being.

Adequate sleep.

Sleep is an extremely effective healing strategy, providing multiple advantages for muscle restoration, cognitive function, and hormonal balance. During sleep, the body creates growth hormone, which aids in tissue repair and muscular development. Seniors should strive for 7-9 hours of quality sleep every night and stick to a consistent sleep routine to increase sleep quality and recovery time.

Nutrition and Hydration

Proper diet and water are essential for the body's recuperation following strength exercise. Seniors should have a well-balanced diet that includes proteins for muscle repair, carbs for energy replenishment, and lipids for inflammation reduction and hormone synthesis. Furthermore, staying hydrated is essential for efficient nutrition transfer and waste disposal. Consuming anti-inflammatory foods, such as omega-3-rich fish, fruits, vegetables, and whole grains, can help with recuperation.

Stress Management

Managing stress is a sometimes ignored element of healing. Chronic stress can impair the body's capacity to recuperate by disrupting sleep quality and hormonal balance. Seniors might reduce stress by practicing deep breathing exercises, meditation, or indulging in pastimes they like. These routines not only help with physical rehabilitation, but also improve mental wellness.

Listen to Your Body

One of the most important tactics for rest and recuperation is to listen to your body. Seniors should pay particular attention to indicators of weariness, discomfort, or pain and adapt their training intensity and rest days as needed. If recuperation is taking longer than expected, it may be time to lower workout intensity, increase rest days, or talk with a healthcare specialist.

Regular Massage and Gentle Stretching

Massage or mild stretching throughout the recuperation phase can help relieve muscular tension and increase flexibility. These techniques can be especially useful for elders, since they improve circulation, reduce muscular pain, and promote relaxation.

Using these rest and recovery measures can considerably improve the efficacy of a strength training program for seniors. Seniors can optimize their physical health, improve their strength training outcomes, and enjoy a higher quality of life by allowing adequate rest time, engaging in active recovery, prioritizing sleep, maintaining proper nutrition and hydration, managing stress, and listening to their bodies' signals.

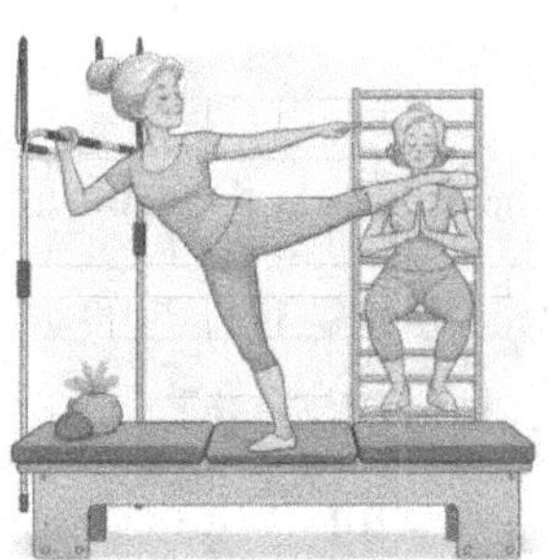

CHAPTER 6

Staying Motivated and Overcoming Challenges

Staying motivated and overcoming challenges are critical aspects of maintaining a strength training regimen, especially for seniors. As individuals age, they may encounter physical limitations, fluctuating motivation levels, and various obstacles that can impede their fitness journey. However, with the right strategies, seniors can sustain their motivation, navigate challenges, and continue to reap the benefits of strength training. Here's a guide on how seniors can stay motivated and overcome common challenges in their strength training journey.

Set Realistic Goals

Setting achievable, realistic goals is foundational for staying motivated. Goals should be specific, measurable, attainable, relevant, and time-bound (SMART). For seniors, goals might range from improving balance and flexibility to increasing muscle strength or reducing joint pain. Achieving these goals provides a sense of accomplishment and motivates seniors to set new challenges.

Celebrate Small Victories

Recognizing and celebrating small victories along the way is crucial for maintaining motivation. Whether it's increasing the weight lifted, completing an extra set, or simply adhering to the workout schedule for a week, acknowledging these achievements provides positive reinforcement and encourages persistence.

Create a Supportive Environment

Having a support system can significantly impact motivation. Friends, family, or fellow seniors engaged in similar fitness routines can offer encouragement, share tips, and celebrate successes together. Joining a group fitness class or online community can also provide a sense of camaraderie and accountability.

Incorporate Variety

Variety in a workout routine can prevent boredom and keep the exercise regimen interesting. Trying different types of strength training exercises, alternating workout locations, or incorporating new activities such as swimming or yoga can rejuvenate interest and motivation. For seniors, variety also ensures a comprehensive approach to fitness, addressing strength, flexibility, balance, and cardiovascular health.

Focus on the Benefits

Reminding oneself of the benefits of strength training can help maintain motivation. Beyond physical improvements, strength training enhances mental health, boosts cognitive function, and promotes independence. Keeping these benefits in mind can motivate seniors to stick with their routine, even when faced with challenges.

Adapt to Physical Limitations

Physical limitations or health issues can pose significant challenges. Adapting the workout routine to accommodate these limitations is key. This might involve modifying exercises, reducing intensity, or incorporating assistive devices. Consulting with healthcare professionals or fitness trainers specialized in senior fitness can provide valuable guidance in making these adjustments.

Manage Expectations

It's important for seniors to manage their expectations regarding progress and outcomes. Physical improvements may occur more slowly compared to younger individuals, and some days may be more challenging than others. Accepting this reality and focusing on consistent effort rather than rapid results can help manage frustration and prevent discouragement.

Establish a Routine

A regular workout schedule can enhance motivation by establishing a routine. Consistency reinforces the habit of exercising, making it a natural part of daily life. For seniors, having a set time and place for workouts can minimize procrastination and make it easier to stay on track.

Seek Inspiration

Finding inspiration from other seniors who are actively engaged in strength training can be incredibly motivating. Success stories, whether from within one's community or found in books, magazines, or online, can provide motivation and proof that it's never too late to improve one's health and fitness.

Staying motivated and overcoming challenges in strength training requires a multifaceted approach, especially for seniors. By setting realistic goals, celebrating small victories, creating a supportive environment, incorporating variety, focusing on the benefits, adapting to physical limitations, managing expectations, establishing a routine, and seeking inspiration, seniors can maintain their motivation, navigate obstacles, and continue to enjoy the myriad benefits of strength training.

Tracking Your Progress

Tracking progress is an essential component of any strength training program, particularly for seniors. It not only gives visible proof of progress, but it also increases motivation, assists in changing training tactics, and guarantees that fitness goals are attained. Here's how seniors may measure their success in strength training:

Set Clear Benchmarks.

Start by setting clear, quantifiable criteria based on your first fitness evaluation and goals. These may include the amount of weight you can lift, the number of repetitions or sets required for a specific activity, balance and flexibility tests, or even how you feel before and after exercises.

Use a workout journal.

Keeping a fitness notebook is a simple yet efficient approach to measure your progress. Each training session should be documented in full, including the exercises performed, weights lifted, sets and reps accomplished, and any differences in how the workouts felt compared to previous sessions. This logbook will eventually give a detailed picture of your development.

Take regular assessments.

Periodic reassessments can assist identify gains in strength, flexibility, balance, and general fitness. Every few months, review the benchmarks established at the start of your program. These assessments may then be used to adjust the training schedule, guaranteeing continual improvement and adaptability to new fitness levels.

Monitor physical and mental changes.

Beyond quantifiable measurements, consider how you feel. Energy levels, sleep quality, mood, and a decrease in joint pain or stiffness are all signs of success. Tracking these improvements might offer a more comprehensive understanding of the effects of your strength training plan.

Celebrate Achievements

Recognize and applaud all successes, no matter how minor. Achieving a personal best, finishing a hard session, or just sticking to your training program are all successes worth celebrating.

Tracking success in strength training is critical for seniors who want to stay motivated, alter their training routines, and achieve long-term fitness objectives. Seniors may stay on track to a better, stronger self by setting goals, keeping a fitness log, conducting regular evaluations, tracking physical and mental improvements, and celebrating accomplishments.

Finding Support and Community

Finding support and community is critical for elders beginning a strength training journey. A supporting network not only motivates and encourages, but it also improves the whole exercise experience by providing guidance, sharing experiences, and creating a sense of belonging. Here's how elders may get support and form a community around their strength training efforts:

Join a fitness group or class.

Many gyms, community centers, and senior groups provide exercise sessions exclusively for older persons. These courses offer a safe, controlled setting for strength training, guided by expert instructors. Furthermore, they provide an excellent opportunity to meet people who have similar fitness objectives and problems.

Participate in online communities.

The internet provides several options for seniors seeking assistance with their fitness quest. Older individuals interested in strength training might find support through online forums, social media groups, and fitness apps. These platforms enable users to exchange suggestions, celebrate accomplishments, and even plan virtual training sessions, creating a feeling of community from the comfort of their own homes.

Find a workout buddy.

Partnering with a friend, family member, or neighbor who shares your health objectives may greatly increase motivation. Workout pals may hold one other responsible, exchange routines, and provide support and encouragement during difficult times.

Engage with Professional Support

Personal trainers or fitness coaches that specialize in senior fitness can give individualized assistance, assisting in the creation of routines that are tailored to individual requirements and goals. They may also provide encouragement and track progress, making strength training more efficient and pleasant.

Volunteer or lead a group.

For individuals who are comfortable in their fitness path, leading a small workout group or offering to assist others with their workouts may be quite fulfilling. Teaching or coaching others not only improves your own knowledge, but it also fosters communal relationships.

Finding support and community is critical for elders participating in strength training. Being part of a supportive network, whether through fitness classes, online forums, exercise partners, professional assistance, or group leadership, may boost motivation, give essential resources, and contribute to a more fun and successful fitness journey.

Adapting to Changes and Staying Committed

Adapting to changes and being dedicated to a strength training plan is critical for seniors, as it assures ongoing improvement and engagement despite the inevitable physical and lifestyle changes that occur with aging. The path to sustaining fitness and health is not straightforward; it needs adaptability, perseverance, and a dedication to self-care.

Embrace flexibility in your routine.

As Elders age, their physical abilities and health circumstances may alter, prompting changes to exercise regimens. It is critical to be willing to adjust exercises, change the intensity, or even move the focus (for example, from strength to flexibility or balance). This adjustability guarantees that your training plan remains in line with your current skills and health requirements.

Set realistic and adjustable goals.

Goals established at the start of your fitness journey may need to be reviewed and altered over time. Setting short-term, attainable objectives can offer a sense of success and incentive to persevere. Reassess and reframe your objectives when circumstances change to ensure they remain attainable and compelling.

Cultivate a positive mindset.

A positive mentality is a valuable tool for overcoming obstacles and maintaining commitment. Celebrate your accomplishments, no matter how minor, and see setbacks as chances to learn and grow. Maintaining a good attitude helps you navigate changes and stay motivated over time.

Seek support and accountability.

Finding a community or support group of like-minded people may offer encouragement, counsel, and a feeling of responsibility. Whether it's family, friends, or other fitness fanatics, having a supporting network may help you stay motivated and adjust to changes easier.

Prioritize consistency above perfection.

Consistency is essential for obtaining the long-term advantages of strength training. Rather of trying for perfection in each session, concentrate on keeping a consistent training regimen. Regular participation, even if it requires altering the intensity or kind of exercise, helps to maintain health and fitness.

To adapt to changes and stay dedicated, seniors must be flexible in their approach, practical in their goal setting, optimistic in their thinking, supported by their community, and focused on consistency. These tactics ensure that elders may continue to get the advantages of strength training while managing changes with perseverance and resolve.

CONCLUSION

As you embark on the wonderful voyage of strength training, "Strength Training for Seniors" will be your constant friend, guiding you to unsurpassed energy and strength, regardless of age. This book is more than simply a compilation of exercises; it exemplifies the force of resilience and the irrefutable spirit of gracefully aging with confidence and health.

Come on a transforming adventure with us. Accept the wisdom, solutions, and support that "Strength Training for Seniors" provides. Let it be your guide as you navigate the challenges and rewards of being active in your senior years. Whether you're a novice or trying to improve your existing practice, this book delivers the tools, inspiration, and insights you need for a successful and rewarding strength training journey.

We encourage you to take the first step toward becoming a better, more vibrant version of yourself. Purchase "Strength Training for Seniors" today to start living a healthier, more active life.

Your travels and experiences are important to us. We would be thrilled if you shared your journey after reading the book and using its techniques in your life. Please consider providing an honest review. Your input not only helps us improve, but it also motivates and guides others in the senior community to take the first step toward their health objectives. Together, let us create a strong, supportive community that demonstrates that strength knows no age.

Embrace change, stay dedicated, and join us in reinventing the aging narrative. "Strength Training for Seniors" is more than simply a book; it's the key to a life in which age is only a number and strength is your constant ally.

Workout Tracker

Week
____

Day
____

Month _______________________

Weekly Goals

- ⬤ ◯ _______________________
- ⬤ ◯ _______________________
- ⬤ ◯ _______________________
- ⬤ ◯ _______________________

Monday Exercises:

Tuesday Exercises:

Wednesday Exercises:

Thursday Exercises:

Friday Exercises:

Saturday Exercises:

Sunday Exercises:

My Motivation

Notes /Reminder

Workout Tracker

Week ___________________

Day ___________________

Month ___________________

Monday Exercises:

Tuesday Exercises:

Wednesday Exercises:

Thursday Exercises:

Friday Exercises:

Saturday Exercises:

Sunday Exercises:

Weekly Goals

- ○ ___________________
- ○ ___________________
- ○ ___________________
- ○ ___________________

My Motivation

Notes /Reminder

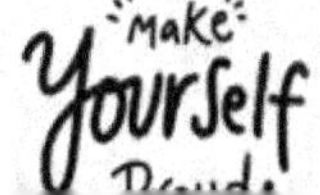

Workout Tracker

Week

Day

Month

Weekly Goals

Monday Exercises:

Tuesday Exercises:

Wednesday Exercises:

Thursday Exercises:

Friday Exercises:

Saturday Exercises:

Sunday Exercises:

My Motivation

Notes /Reminder

Make Yourself Proud

Workout Tracker

Week ________________________

Day ________________________

Month ________________________

Monday Exercises:

Weekly Goals

- ☐ ________________________
- ☐ ________________________
- ☐ ________________________
- ☐ ________________________

Tuesday Exercises:

Wednesday Exercises:

My Motivation

Thursday Exercises:

Friday Exercises:

Notes /Reminder

Saturday Exercises:

Sunday Exercises:

Workout Tracker

Week _______________________

Day _______________________

Month _______________________

Monday Exercises:

Tuesday Exercises:

Wednesday Exercises:

Thursday Exercises:

Friday Exercises:

Saturday Exercises:

Sunday Exercises:

Weekly Goals

- ☐ _______________________
- ☐ _______________________
- ☐ _______________________
- ☐ _______________________

My Motivation

Notes /Reminder

Workout Tracker

Week _______________________

Day _______________________

Month _______________________

Weekly Goals

- ⬤ ☐ ....
- ⬤ ☐ ....
- ⬤ ☐ ....
- ⬤ ☐ ....

Monday Exercises:

Tuesday Exercises:

Wednesday Exercises:

Thursday Exercises:

Friday Exercises:

Saturday Exercises:

Sunday Exercises:

My Motivation

Notes /Reminder

Workout Tracker

Week ______________________

Day ______________________

Month ______________________

Weekly Goals

○ ....
○ ....
○ ....
○ ....

Monday Exercises:

Tuesday Exercises:

Wednesday Exercises:

Thursday Exercises:

My Motivation

Friday Exercises:

Notes /Reminder

Saturday Exercises:

Sunday Exercises:

Make
Yourself
. Proud .

Workout Tracker

Week

Day

Month

Weekly Goals

Monday Exercises:

Tuesday Exercises:

Wednesday Exercises:

My Motivation

Thursday Exercises:

Friday Exercises:

Notes /Reminder

Saturday Exercises:

Sunday Exercises:

Workout Tracker

Week

Day

Month

Weekly Goals

- ☐
- ☐
- ☐
- ☐

Monday Exercises:

Tuesday Exercises:

Wednesday Exercises:

My Motivation

Thursday Exercises:

Friday Exercises:

Notes /Reminder

Saturday Exercises:

Sunday Exercises:

Workout Tracker

Week ___________________

Day ___________________

Month ___________________

Monday Exercises:

Tuesday Exercises:

Wednesday Exercises:

Thursday Exercises:

Friday Exercises:

Saturday Exercises:

Sunday Exercises:

Weekly Goals

- ☐ ___________________
- ☐ ___________________
- ☐ ___________________
- ☐ ___________________

My Motivation

Notes /Reminder

Workout Tracker

Week

Day

Month

Monday Exercises:

Weekly Goals

Tuesday Exercises:

Wednesday Exercises:

My Motivation

Thursday Exercises:

Friday Exercises:

Notes /Reminder

Saturday Exercises:

Sunday Exercises:

Workout Tracker

Week

Day

Month

Weekly Goals

Monday Exercises:

Tuesday Exercises:

Wednesday Exercises:

Thursday Exercises:

My Motivation

Friday Exercises:

Notes /Reminder

Saturday Exercises:

Sunday Exercises:

Workout Tracker

Week

Day

Month

Monday Exercises:

Tuesday Exercises:

Weekly Goals

- [ ] ....
- [ ] ....
- [ ] ....
- [ ] ....

Wednesday Exercises:

My Motivation

Thursday Exercises:

Friday Exercises:

Notes /Reminder

Saturday Exercises:

Sunday Exercises: